Ancient remedies revived

How timeless Ancient Healing Traditions Can Transform Your Health

J. Waller

© [2024] J. Waller. All rights reserved.

No part of this book may be reproduced, distributed, or transmitted in any form or by any means, including photocopying, recording, or other electronic or mechanical methods, without the prior written permission of the author, except in the case of brief quotations embodied in critical reviews and certain other noncommercial uses permitted by copyright law.

INTRODUCTION 5
    The Renewal of Ancient Healing Practices in Modern Health 5

CHAPTER ONE: THE FOUNDATIONS OF ANCIENT HEALING 12
    Historical Context for Ancient Healing Traditions 12

CHAPTER 2: KEY HERBS AND THEIR USES 22
    Introduction to Key Medicinal Herbs Used in Ancient Traditions 22

CHAPTER 3: KEY HERBS AND THEIR USES. 35
    Introduction to Key Medicinal Herbs Used in Ancient Traditions 35

CHAPTER 4: KEY HERBS AND THEIR APPLICATIONS 48
    Introduction to Key Medicinal Herbs Used in Ancient Traditions 48

CHAPTER 5: ANCIENT DIETARY PRACTICES FOR HEALTH. 55
    The Role of Diet in Ancient Healing Systems 55

CHAPTER 6: MIND-BODY CONNECTION. 68
    Understanding the Importance of Mental Health in Ancient Healing 68

CHAPTER 7: RITUALS AND REMEDIES FOR COMMON AILS. 80
    Solutions for Common Issues 80

CHAPTER 8: THE ROLE OF SPIRITUALITY IN HEALING 93
    The Connection Between Spirituality and Health 93

CHAPTER 9: MODERN APPLICATION OF ANCIENT WISDOM 102
    Ethical Concerns and Sustainability in Sourcing Natural Remedies 102

CHAPTER 10: A PRACTICAL GUIDE TO BEGINNING YOUR HEALING JOURNEY. **106**

    Creating Your Personal Healing Plan 106

CONCLUSION: REVITALIZING ANCIENT WISDOM FOR MODERN WELLNESS. **116**

THE END **124**

Introduction

In our fast-paced, modern society, when stress and chronic illnesses are common, many people seek solace in the wisdom of the past. The revival of traditional healing methods is more than a fad; it is a significant return to the roots of holistic health, emphasizing the interdependence of body, mind, and spirit. This book, "Ancient Remedies Revived: How Timeless Ancient Healing Traditions Can Transform Your Health," is intended to take you on a trip through the rich tapestry of old healing traditions, exposing how these time-tested remedies can benefit your well-being in the modern world.

The Renewal of Ancient Healing Practices in Modern Health

The growing interest in traditional medicines is more than just nostalgia for simpler times. It reflects a growing understanding of the limitations of conventional medicine, which frequently treats symptoms rather than addressing underlying causes. According to a 2021 poll by the National Center for alternative and Integrative Health, approximately 38% of adults in the United States reported utilizing some type of alternative health strategy, including herbal remedies, yoga, and meditation.

This shift to integrative health techniques has paved the way for a revival of historic practices.

The COVID-19 epidemic has served as a spark for this movement, causing people to reconsider their health strategies. People are looking for ways to enhance their immune systems and improve their overall health, leading them to investigate ancient traditions anchored in nature and time-honored wisdom.

As we manage a world riddled with uncertainties and health issues, ancient civilizations' teachings can provide helpful insights. For ages, cultures such as Traditional Chinese Medicine, Ayurveda, and Indigenous healing traditions have refined their methodologies, providing a wealth of information that can be applied today.

Importance of Integrating Traditional Remedies Into Modern Lifestyles

In a society where convenience frequently trumps mindfulness, it's tempting to underestimate the effectiveness of natural therapies. However, incorporating traditional treatments into our daily lives can result in a more holistic and sustainable approach to health. Herbal therapies, for example, can provide a gentler but equally effective alternative to prescription drugs for treating common problems such as anxiety, inflammation, and digestive disorders. A study published in the Journal of Ethnopharmacology revealed that many herbs traditionally utilized for their medicinal characteristics have scientifically verified benefits, making them worthy of our attention.

Incorporating these traditional methods into our life does not mean abandoning contemporary medicine, but rather fostering a harmonious balance between the two. Individuals can develop a more comprehensive awareness of their health by combining traditional and alternative treatments. For example, practicing mindfulness meditation or yoga can supplement medical therapies for chronic diseases, boosting emotional resilience and promoting physical well-being.

Furthermore, as we become more mindful of environmental sustainability, ancient treatments can present a more environmentally responsible option than manufactured equivalents. Traditional techniques stress the use of locally sourced herbs and natural materials, building a connection with the environment that many modern health approaches neglect.

An overview of what readers might expect from this book

In "Ancient Remedies Revived," readers will embark on a fascinating journey through ancient healing techniques that have weathered the test of time. The book is divided into sections, each meant to provide a thorough grasp of the concepts, practices, and prospects of these treatments.

Beginning with a thorough examination of the historical backdrop of ancient healing methods, we will uncover the rich legacies of cultures such as Ayurveda, Traditional Chinese Medicine, and Indigenous healing. Understanding the origins of these traditions will allow readers to recognize their importance in today's environment.

Next, we'll look at the most effective herbs and their applications, including profiles of time-honored botanicals that can be simply integrated into daily routines. Readers of all skill levels will benefit from practical advice on how to prepare and use these herbs.

Furthermore, the book will delve into traditional dietary habits that promote health and vitality, introducing readers to recipes inspired by these traditions. From fermented meals to herbal infusions, these culinary traditions will nourish the body while also pleasing the senses.

Mind-body activities will also take center stage, emphasizing the significance of mental and emotional well-being in overall health. Readers will be given techniques for mindfulness, meditation, and other spiritual practices to help them establish a deeper connection with themselves.

Each chapter will feature practical cures for common ailments, as well as anecdotal success stories that demonstrate the ancient traditions' transformational potential. Readers will be encouraged and inspired as they learn how others have healed and prospered by implementing these methods.

Finally, we'll look at modern applications of ancient wisdom, demonstrating how practitioners are successfully incorporating these cures into their practices. This section will illustrate not just the efficacy of these approaches, but also the significance of responsible sourcing and ethical considerations.

As we read through the pages of "Ancient Remedies Revived," we will obtain not just knowledge but also practical methods for improving our health and well-being. The goal is to spark a movement toward a more balanced, aware, and harmonious approach to health—one that acknowledges our ancestors' wisdom while welcoming the opportunities of the present.

Are you prepared to learn the ageless techniques of traditional healing? Join us on this transforming journey to reconnect with the earth's riches and revitalize our health with ancient wisdom.

Chapter One: The Foundations of Ancient Healing

Historical Context for Ancient Healing Traditions

Since the birth of civilization, humans have strived to comprehend and combat sickness. In a world where medical science as we know it did not exist, ancient peoples relied on nature and their observations of the human body to develop healing methods that not only treated physical ailments but also promoted general well-being. Ancient healing traditions have thousands of years of history, and they are frequently connected with the spiritual and cultural beliefs of the communities who practice them.

In ancient Egypt, for example, medicine was inextricably intertwined with religion. Priests served as both healers and mediators between the gods and the people. They used a variety of therapies, from herbal treatments to surgical techniques, which were frequently accompanied by incantations and rituals to elicit heavenly favor. Similarly, ancient Greece set the framework for most of Western medicine through figures such as Hippocrates, also known as the "Father of Medicine." Hippocrates emphasized the necessity of watching patients and their surroundings, pioneering a method of diagnosis that is still appreciated today.

As civilizations advanced, so did their knowledge of health. Ayurveda emerged in India circa 1500 BCE, introducing a holistic system that emphasized equilibrium between the body, mind, and spirit. Similarly, Traditional Chinese Medicine (TCM), which has over 2,500 years of history, incorporates the ideas of balance and harmony, promoting health through procedures such as acupuncture, herbal medicines, and dietary habits.

As communities matured, their healing techniques grew more organized. Ancient books, such as China's Huangdi Neijing (Yellow Emperor's Inner Canon) and India's Charaka Samhita, gathered information and ways to preserve these traditions for future generations. Such books addressed not just the therapies themselves, but also the philosophy underlying them, demonstrating how health and spirituality were connected in ancient times.

Major Cultures: Their Contributions

Traditional Chinese medicine (TCM)

Traditional Chinese Medicine is one of the oldest holistic health care systems still in use today. It is based on the idea of Qi (pronounced "chee"), the essential life force that circulates throughout the body via paths known as meridians. TCM sees health as a harmonious balance of Yin and Yang, the two forces that exist in everything. When these factors are out of balance, sickness can develop.

TCM places a strong emphasis on practices such as acupuncture and herbal treatment. Acupuncture involves placing small needles into certain places on the body to encourage the flow of Qi, which promotes healing and relieves pain. Herbal treatments, which are frequently made from a combination of plants, minerals, and animal products, are personalized to each patient depending on their specific conditions and overall constitution.

In addition to acupuncture and herbal therapy, TCM incorporates techniques like Tai Chi and Qigong, which emphasize gentle movement and breath control to improve physical and mental health. These practices are more than just exercises; they are firmly anchored in philosophical notions and help the practitioner connect with the universe's forces.

Ayurveda

Ayurveda, which originated in India, is one of the world's oldest medical systems, dating back over 5,000 years. The title "Ayurveda" means "the science of life," and its principles emphasize the harmony of the body, mind, and spirit. Ayurveda recognizes three major energies or doshas: vata, pitta, and kapha, which are thought to influence physical and mental functions.

Ayurvedic practitioners examine an individual's dosha before recommending specific dietary and lifestyle adjustments, herbal supplements, and panchakarma cleansing methods. This holistic approach promotes patients to understand their own constitutions and how they interact with their surroundings, improving health and preventing disease via self-awareness.

Ayurveda also emphasizes digestion and metabolism, claiming that a robust digestive system is essential for general health. Herbal treatments, such as turmeric for inflammation and ginger for digestion, are essential to Ayurvedic procedures and are frequently prepared in methods that increase their medicinal powers.

Indigenous Healing Practices.

Indigenous civilizations all around the world have evolved extensive healing traditions based on their relationship to the land and nature. These techniques frequently entail a thorough grasp of the local flora and wildlife, which is passed down through generations. For example, Native American healing traditions take a holistic approach to health that includes physical, emotional, and spiritual well-being.

Indigenous societies' traditional healing techniques frequently include ceremonies, rituals, and the usage of medicinal herbs. Many Indigenous healers are spiritual leaders who use prayer, music, and dance to channel healing energies. These practices also emphasize the sense of community, with group gatherings playing an important role in the healing process.

In Australia, Aboriginal healing methods include the use of bush medicine, which makes use of local flora' therapeutic characteristics. These cures, when combined with storytelling and cultural activities, constitute a comprehensive strategy that connects individuals to their heritage and environment.

Principles of Holistic Health in Traditional Practices

The concept of holistic health is central to ancient healing practices. Unlike traditional Western medicine, which frequently focuses primarily on the physical body, holistic health recognizes the interdependence of body, mind, and spirit. This approach understands that emotional and spiritual health have a substantial impact on physical well-being.

Interconnectedness between the body and mind

Ancient healing traditions have continuously emphasized the interconnectedness of the mind and body. Emotions can emerge as physical problems, so addressing mental health is critical for total wellness. For example, Ayurveda believes that stress and bad emotions can upset the equilibrium of doshas, resulting in sickness. Similarly, TCM recognizes the importance of emotional well-being in sustaining the flow of Qi, and activities like as meditation and mindfulness are critical to maintaining mental equilibrium.

Individualized treatments

Another important aspect of ancient healing is the emphasis on personalized care. Practitioners acknowledge that each individual has unique physical, emotional, and spiritual needs. This approach is evident in both TCM and Ayurveda, where therapies are personalized to each individual depending on their unique constitution and circumstances. Ancient healing traditions encourage long-term health and vitality by focusing on the full person rather than just the symptoms.

Prevention and Lifestyle Choices

Ancient therapeutic practices frequently emphasize prevention rather than reaction. They promote healthy lifestyle choices such as food, physical activity, and stress management approaches. For example, Ayurvedic methods promote a balanced diet based on an individual's dosha and the seasons, whereas TCM emphasizes seasonal eating and adapting one's lifestyle to natural cycles.

Connection with Nature

Finally, ancient healing traditions are profoundly linked to nature. This connection is expressed through the use of natural treatments, awareness of environmental cycles, and the conviction that the soil contains all needed for health and healing. Individuals who cultivate a bond with the natural world can tap into its curative capabilities, which ancient cultures innately recognized.

Ancient healing traditions lay the groundwork for a rich and diverse body of knowledge that has the potential to revolutionize our understanding of health and wellness. Exploring the historical settings and contributions of other civilizations allows us to comprehend the depth of wisdom buried in these traditions. By embracing the ideas of holistic health—interconnectedness, tailored treatment, preventive, and a connection to nature—we can incorporate these traditional solutions into our modern lives, paving the path for a healthier, more balanced future.

Chapter 2: Key Herbs and their Uses

Introduction to Key Medicinal Herbs Used in Ancient Traditions

As we investigate the historical practices that have impacted our concept of health, we cannot ignore the importance of therapeutic herbs. For millennia, societies all over the world have used plants to cure, nourish, and restore balance to the body and mind. These herbs are more than just ingredients; they exemplify humanity's relationship with nature and its wisdom.

This chapter exposes you to some of the most important medicinal herbs used in ancient traditions, highlighting their astonishing advantages and how they can be easily integrated into our modern life. From the vivid color of turmeric to the pungent flavor of ginger, each herb has a healing tradition that lives on today.

Let's look at the profiles of 10-15 major herbs, discovering their historic usage, active ingredients, and the best ways to prepare and incorporate them into our daily lives.

Profiles of Key Herb

Turmeric (Curcuma Longa)

Turmeric, also known as the "golden spice," has been used in Ayurvedic and Traditional Chinese medicine (TCM) for ages. Its main active ingredient, curcumin, is well-known for its powerful anti-inflammatory and antioxidant capabilities. Turmeric is frequently used to promote joint health, improve digestive function, and treat skin issues.

Preparation and incorporation:

Golden Milk: Mix turmeric powder into warm milk (dairy or plant-based) and sweeten with honey. Add a sprinkle of black pepper to improve absorption.

Sprinkle turmeric on roasted veggies, soups, or curries to enhance flavor and health benefits.

Ginger (zingiber officinale)

Ginger has been utilized in numerous cultures for millennia and is revered for its ability to improve digestion and relieve nausea. It functions as a natural anti-inflammatory and helps to manage pain, especially in disorders like osteoarthritis.

Preparation and incorporation:

Ginger Tea: Slice fresh ginger and soak in boiling water for 10 minutes. Add lemon and honey to taste.

Grate ginger into stir-fries, marinades, or baked products to add a fiery flavor and health benefits.

Ashwagandha (Withania somnifera).

Ashwagandha, a potent adaptogen, has long been acclaimed in Ayurveda for its ability to alleviate stress and anxiety while increasing overall vigor. Its bioactive components, including withanolides, help to regulate cortisol levels and boost energy.

Preparation and incorporation:

Powdered Supplement: Add ashwagandha powder to smoothies or porridge.

Infuse ashwagandha in hot water to make a relaxing tea before bedtime.

Holy Basil (Ocimum Sanctum)

Holy basil, also known as Tulsi, is a sacred herb in India that is appreciated for its adaptogenic and anti-inflammatory effects. It strengthens the immune system and improves mental clarity.

Preparation and incorporation:

Holy Basil Tea: To make a fragrant tea, steep fresh or dried leaves in boiling water.

Holy basil can be used as a garnish in a variety of foods, including salads and soups.

Garlic (Allium sativum).

Garlic, a potent antibacterial and immune-boosting herb, has long been used in various cultures for its health advantages. It is especially effective against infections and promotes cardiovascular health.

Preparation and incorporation:

Crush raw garlic and add it to salad dressings or spreads.

Culinary Use: Sauté garlic in olive oil to provide flavor to a variety of recipes.

Peppermint (Mentha Piperita)

This fragrant plant is well-known for its relaxing effects on the digestive tract. Peppermint oil has also been investigated for its potential to alleviate headaches and tension.

Preparation and incorporation:

Brew fresh peppermint leaves in hot water for a delightful tea.

Peppermint can be used as a garnish in cocktails, salads, and desserts.

Cinnamon (Cinnamomum Verum)

Cinnamon, known for its pleasant flavor and scent, has long been utilized in traditional medicine for its antioxidant and anti-inflammatory properties. It can help manage blood sugar and promote heart health.

Preparation and incorporation:

Cinnamon Spice Mix: Sprinkle ground cinnamon over porridge, smoothies, or baked goods.

Cinnamon Tea: Steep a cinnamon stick in hot water for a calming beverage.

Echinacea (Echinacea Purpurea)

Echinacea, a native North American herb, is largely used to stimulate the immune system and treat respiratory infections. Its active components may assist to shorten the duration of colds and flu.

Preparation and incorporation:

To make echinacea tea, steep dried echinacea blossoms in hot water.

Tinctures: Use echinacea extracts during the cold and flu season.

Ginseng (panax ginseng)

Ginseng, a potent adaptogen, has long been revered in Traditional Chinese Medicine for its energy-boosting and immune-enhancing effects. It may aid to boost cognitive function and minimize weariness.

Preparation and incorporation:

Ginseng Tea: Steep slices of ginseng root in boiling water.

Supplement Form: Use ginseng extract or capsules as directed.

Nettles (Urtica dioica)

Nettle, commonly referred to be a weed, is a nutritious powerhouse high in vitamins and minerals. It is typically used to promote urinary health and reduce inflammation.

Preparation and incorporation:

Steep dried nettle leaves in boiling water to make a nutritious tea.

Culinary Use: Sauté young nettle leaves in olive oil for a healthful side dish.

Milk thistle (silybum marianum)

Milk thistle, known for its liver-protective characteristics, has been used for generations to help with detoxification and liver function. Its active ingredient, silymarin, is credited with these properties.

Preparation and incorporation:

Milk Thistle Tea: To make a cleansing tea, steep the seeds in hot water.

Capsules or Tinctures: Available in a variety of supplement forms to support the liver.

Fenugreek (Trigonella foenum-graecum).

This plant has long been used to aid digestion and milk production in nursing women. It may also assist to control blood sugar levels.

Preparation and incorporation:

Fenugreek Tea: Steep seeds in hot water for a healthy beverage.

Fenugreek leaves or seeds can be added to curries and stews to enhance flavor and provide health benefits.

Sage (salvia officinalis)

Sage is well-known for its culinary uses, but it also has antibacterial and anti-inflammatory qualities. It may help with digestion difficulties and promote cognitive wellness.

Preparation and incorporation:

Sage Tea: Make a calming beverage by infusing dried leaves in hot water.

Use sage in stuffings, sauces, and roasted meals.

Dandelions (Taraxacum officinale)

Dandelion, a weed that is commonly regarded as a nuisance, has a long history of medicinal applications. Its leaves and roots are used to promote liver function and detoxification.

Ancient remedies revived

Preparation and incorporation:

Dandelion Tea: Steep dried dandelion roots or leaves in boiling water.

Young dandelion greens can be added to salads to increase their nutritional value.

Melissa officinalis, or lemon balm

Lemon balm, a member of the mint family, is known for its relaxing properties and capacity to treat anxiety and sleeplessness.

Preparation and incorporation:

Steep fresh or dried lemon balm leaves in boiling water to make a calming tea.

Add lemon balm to desserts, salads, or cocktails.

How to Prepare and Use These Herbs in Your Daily Life

Including herbs in your everyday routine can be both simple and gratifying. Here are some practical instructions for preparing and using these medicinal plants.

Infusions and teas:

Making herbal teas or infusions is one of the most convenient ways to absorb therapeutic herbs. Simply immerse the dried leaves, blossoms, or roots in boiling water for 5–15 minutes, depending on the herb. Strain, and enjoy. Consider combining different herbs to create a unique brew that addresses specific health concerns.

Tinctures and extracts:

Herbal tinctures are concentrated liquid extracts produced by soaking herbs in alcohol or vinegar. They provide an effective technique to gain the advantages of herbs in tiny amounts. Follow the dose recommendations and seek help from a healthcare expert.

Powders:

Many herbs, like turmeric and ashwagandha, can be eaten in powdered form. Add them to smoothies, yogurt, or porridge. You can also make herbal blends for specific health benefits, like a morning energy boost or a relaxing evening regimen.

Cooking:

Adding herbs to your culinary range not only enhances

Chapter 3: Key Herbs and Their Uses.

Introduction to Key Medicinal Herbs Used in Ancient Traditions

Throughout history, cultures have relied largely on nature's wisdom to solve health concerns and improve well-being. As we journey into the realm of traditional healing traditions, medicinal herbs play an important role that cannot be overlooked. These plants, with their complex profiles of active chemicals and extraordinary advantages, have served as the foundation for a variety of medicinal methods.

The usage of plants has a long history, stretching back to India's Ayurvedic literature and Indigenous nations' herbal traditions. Their applications range from simple home cures to complex pharmaceutical treatments. While modern medicine has made significant advances, the renewed interest in these age-old cures provides a rare opportunity for anyone seeking natural and holistic approaches to health.

In this chapter, we will look at major herbs' historical significance, medical characteristics, and practical applications. By restoring ancient herbs into our modern lives, we can use their healing properties to improve our daily routines and general health.

Profiles of Key Herb

Turmeric (Curcuma Longa)

Turmeric, also known as the "golden spice," has been valued in Ayurvedic and Traditional Chinese medicine (TCM) for millennia. Curcumin, its principal active component, is a potent anti-inflammatory drug that has received attention in recent scientific studies for its capacity to promote joint health and treat chronic disorders.

Preparation and incorporation:

Golden Milk: Combine turmeric powder with warm milk (dairy or plant-based) and sweeten with honey. A sprinkle of black pepper can dramatically improve curcumin absorption.

Sprinkle turmeric in soups, curries, or roasted veggies to add taste and health benefits.

Ginger (zingiber officinale)

Ginger, a popular spice in many cuisines, has been known for its digestive advantages and capacity to alleviate nausea. Its anti-inflammatory effects make it very useful for treating arthritis and other inflammatory diseases.

Preparation and incorporation:

Ginger Tea: Slice fresh ginger and soak in boiling water for about 10 minutes, adding lemon and honey to taste.

Culinary Use: Grate ginger into stir-fries, smoothies, or baked goods to add a fiery kick and numerous health benefits.

Ashwagandha (Withania somnifera).

This strong adaptogen has long been used in Ayurvedic medicine for its stress-relieving qualities. Ashwagandha helps to balance cortisol levels, which promotes mental clarity and emotional stability.

Preparation and incorporation:

Powdered Supplement: Add ashwagandha powder to smoothies or porridge for a nutritional boost.

Herbal Tea: Infuse ashwagandha in hot water for a relaxing drink, especially before bedtime.

Holy Basil (Ocimum Sanctum)

Holy basil, commonly known as Tulsi, is revered in Hindu culture and appreciated for its adaptogenic characteristics. It strengthens the immune system and helps to regulate stress and anxiety.

Preparation and incorporation:

Holy Basil Tea: To make a fragrant herbal tea, steep fresh or dried leaves in boiling water.

Use holy basil in salads, soups, or as a garnish to enhance flavor and health benefits.

Garlic (Allium sativum).

Garlic, a potent antibacterial, has a long history of use in traditional medicine to enhance immunity and treat infections. Its cardiovascular effects, including blood pressure management, make it an indispensable herb in many diets.

Preparation and incorporation:

Raw Consumption: Crush raw garlic and put it into salad dressings or dips for a nutritious boost.

Culinary Application: Sauté garlic in olive oil as a base for many recipes to improve flavor and nutrients.

Peppermint (Mentha Piperita)

Peppermint is well-known for its refreshing flavor and ability to ease stomach disorders and tension headaches.

Preparation and incorporation:

Peppermint Tea: Brew fresh leaves in hot water for a relaxing drink.

For a refreshing twist, try adding peppermint to desserts, salads, or cocktails.

Cinnamon (Cinnamomum Verum)

This pungent spice is known for its antioxidant effects and capacity to manage blood sugar levels. Cinnamon can improve digestive health and has been demonstrated to have anti-inflammatory properties.

Preparation and incorporation:

Cinnamon Spice Mix: Add ground cinnamon to porridge, smoothies, or baked goods for extra flavor and health benefits.

Cinnamon Tea: Steep a cinnamon stick in hot water for a calming beverage.

Echinacea (Echinacea Purpurea)

Echinacea, a well-known immune booster, is frequently used to treat the onset of colds and flu. Its components may aid in reducing the length and severity of respiratory infections.

Preparation and incorporation:

Echinacea Tea: For a therapeutic infusion, steep dried echinacea blossoms in hot water.

Tinctures: Use echinacea extracts to stay healthy during the cold and flu season.

Ginseng (panax ginseng)

Ginseng, which is revered for its stimulating benefits, has been used in traditional Chinese medicine for millennia to improve stamina and cognitive performance. Its adaptogenic properties enable the body to withstand stress.

Preparation and incorporation:

Ginseng Tea: To make a refreshing drink, steep slices of ginseng root in hot water.

Supplement Form: Available in extracts or capsules; follow your healthcare provider's dose recommendations.

Nettles (Urtica dioica)

Often dismissed as a plant, nettle is a nutritious powerhouse rich in vitamins and minerals. It has long been used for its anti-inflammatory effects and to promote urinary health.

Preparation and incorporation:

Steep dried nettle leaves in boiling water to create a nutrient-rich infusion.

Cooking Tip: Sauté fresh nettle leaves in olive oil for a tasty side dish.

Milk thistle (silybum marianum)

Milk thistle, known for its liver-protective properties, has been utilized for generations to help the body's detoxification processes.

Preparation and incorporation:

Milk Thistle Tea: Brew dry seeds in hot water to make a cleaning beverage.

Capsules and tinctures are available in a variety of formats to assist liver function.

Fenugreek (Trigonella foenum-graecum).

This herb has been traditionally used to aid digestion and lactation in nursing moms. Its components may help control blood sugar levels.

Preparation and incorporation:

Fenugreek Tea: Steep seeds in hot water for a healthy beverage.

Fenugreek leaves or seeds can be added to curries and stews to enhance flavor and provide health benefits.

Sage (salvia officinalis)

Sage is well-known for its culinary uses, but it also has antibacterial and antiinflammatory effects. It may improve intestinal health and cognitive function.

Preparation and incorporation:

Sage Tea: Make a calming drink by infusing dried leaves in hot water.

Use sage in stuffing, sauces, or roasted meats to add taste and health benefits.

Dandelions (Taraxacum officinale)

Dandelions, which are frequently rejected as weeds, have a long history of usage in herbal medicine due to their cleansing characteristics and capacity to improve liver health.

Preparation and incorporation:

Dandelion Tea: To make a refreshing beverage, steep dried roots or leaves in hot water.

Young dandelion greens make a healthful complement to salads.

Melissa officinalis, or lemon balm

This fragrant plant is well-known for its soothing properties, which are frequently used to relieve anxiety and induce relaxation.

Preparation and incorporation:

Lemon Balm Tea: To make a calming drink, steep fresh or dried leaves in hot water.

Lemon balm can be used in desserts, salads, and cocktails to add a refreshing flavor.

How to Prepare and Use These Herbs in Your Daily Life

Incorporating herbs into your daily routine can be both beneficial and simple. Here are some practical instructions for preparing and using these therapeutic plants effectively:

Infusions and teas:

Making herbal teas is a simple and effective way to absorb therapeutic herbs. Steep dried plants, flowers, or roots in boiling water for a few minutes to extract their therapeutic ingredients. Consider combining several herbs to create a customized infusion that addresses specific health requirements.

Tinctures and extracts:

Herbal tinctures are concentrated extracts made from soaking herbs in alcohol or vinegar. They provide an effective technique to ingest herbs in modest dosages. Follow the dosage guidelines carefully, and if you are unclear, see a healthcare expert.

Powders:

Many herbs can be taken in powdered form, making them easy to incorporate into smoothies, yogurt, or porridge. Experiment with combining herbs to achieve specific health goals, such as an invigorating morning beverage or a relaxing evening routine.

Chapter 4: Key Herbs and Their Applications

Introduction to Key Medicinal Herbs Used in Ancient Traditions

Medicinal herbs have played an important role in healing techniques across countries and time periods. From Ayurveda and Traditional Chinese Medicine to Indigenous herbal traditions, these plants have bioactive substances that have been used to treat health issues and improve well-being. In today's modern society, there is a growing interest in natural therapies as a way to achieve holistic health.

This chapter delves into the histories of major herbs, their therapeutic characteristics, and practical uses. By incorporating these herbs into our daily lives, we may harness their healing power and embrace a more natural approach to maintaining our health.

Profiles of Key Herb

Turmeric (Curcuma Longa)

Benefits: Anti-inflammatory, promotes joint health, and increases immunity.

Uses include golden milk, soups, and curries.

Ginger (zingiber officinale)

Benefits: Improves digestion, relieves nausea, and is anti-inflammatory.

Uses include ginger tea, stir-fries, and baked products.

Ashwagandha (Withania somnifera).

Benefits: Lowers stress, improves mental clarity, and promotes adrenal health.

Uses include smoothies and herbal tea.

Holy Basil (Ocimum Sanctum)

Benefits: Reduces stress and anxiety, and increases immunity.

Uses include herbal tea and salads.

Garlic (Allium sativum).

effects include antimicrobial, immune-boosting, and cardiovascular effects.

Uses: Raw in dressings and sautéed in meals.

Peppermint (Mentha Piperita)

Benefits: Treats stomach problems and improves headaches.

Uses include peppermint tea and sweets.

Cinnamon (Cinnamomum Verum)

Benefits include antioxidant activity, blood sugar regulation, and digestive assistance.

Uses include baked items, oatmeal, and cinnamon tea.

Echinacea (Echinacea Purpurea)

Benefits: Increases immunity and may shorten cold duration.

Uses: Echinacea tea and tinctures.

Ginseng (panax ginseng)

Benefits: Energizes and improves cognitive function.

Uses: Ginseng tea and pills.

Nettles (Urtica dioica)

Benefits: Anti-inflammatory; improves urinary health.

Uses: Nettle tea and sautéed greens.

Milk thistle (silybum marianum)

Benefits: Promotes liver health and cleansing.

Uses: Milk thistle tea and capsules.

Fenugreek (Trigonella foenum-graecum).

Benefits: Improves digestion, promotes lactation, and controls blood sugar.

Uses: Fenugreek tea and curries.

Sage (salvia officinalis)

Benefits: Antimicrobial; improves cognitive function.

Uses include sage tea, stuffing, and sauces.

Dandelions (Taraxacum officinale)

Benefits: Detoxifies and promotes liver health.

Uses: Dandelion tea and salads.

Melissa officinalis, or lemon balm

Benefits: Calming, reduces anxiety.

Lemon balm tea can be used in desserts.

How to Prepare and Use These Herbs in Your Daily Life

Incorporating medicinal plants into daily practices can be simple and fun.

Infusions & Teas: Make herbal tea by steeping dry herbs in hot water to extract therapeutic components.

Tinctures and Extracts: For maximum impact, use concentrated herbal extracts and adhere to dosage guidelines.

Powders: Add powdered herbs to smoothies, cereal, or yogurt to boost nutrition.

Cooking: Incorporate fresh or dried herbs into various foods to boost flavor and health benefits.

Integrating these herbs into daily activities allows people to reap the health advantages while also appreciating the rich flavors and traditions they bring.

Ancient remedies revived

Chapter 5: Ancient Dietary Practices for Health.

The Role of Diet in Ancient Healing Systems

Diet has been important to human health and well-being since the dawn of civilization. Ancient cultures recognized that the foods they ate may have a significant impact on their physical and mental health. While contemporary medicine frequently focuses on treating symptoms, ancient healing systems acknowledged the value of a well-balanced diet as a foundation for avoiding sickness and increasing longevity.

Hippocrates famously declared in ancient Greece, "Let food be thy medicine and medicine be thy food." This idea spread throughout civilizations, emphasizing the relationship between diet and health.

Food, according to Traditional Chinese Medicine (TCM), is more than just sustenance; it is also a potent instrument for preserving physiological equilibrium. Similarly, Ayurvedic teachings in India highlight the need of eating according to one's constitution, or dosha, implying that food may heal and restore balance.

Dietary practices are recognized as an important component of health and healing across civilizations. For example, the Native American approach frequently included seasonal eating and the use of local, complete foods, whereas Mediterranean diets stressed fruits, vegetables, whole grains, and healthy fats. These customs serve as a reminder that our eating habits have an impact on everything from our energy levels to our emotional health.

Common Dietary Practices and Health Benefits

Fermented foods

Fermentation is one of the oldest techniques of food preservation, converting raw materials into probiotic-rich sources of nutrients. Ancient societies, including the Chinese with fermented soy products and the Koreans with kimchi, understood the health benefits of fermented foods.

Health Benefits:

Gut Health: Fermented foods contain helpful microorganisms that help with digestion and nutrition absorption.

Enhanced Immunity: A healthy gut microbiome is directly linked to a strong immune system, which aids in illness prevention.

Fermentation breaks down antinutrients, increasing vitamin and mineral bioavailability.

Examples:

Sauerkraut is finely shredded cabbage fermented with lactic acid bacteria.

Kefir is a fermented milk drink high in probiotics.

Fasting

Fasting has long been practiced in many cultures and religions, and it is frequently seen as a spiritual practice. Ancient Egyptians, Greeks, and Ayurvedic practitioners believed that fasting allowed the body to purify and recover.

Health Benefits:

Cellular Repair: Fasting induces autophagy, a process by which cells eliminate damaged components and renew.

Intermittent fasting can help with insulin sensitivity and weight management.

Mental Clarity: Many people find that fasting improves their mental clarity and attention.

Examples:

Intermittent fasting refers to cycles of eating and fasting, such as the 16/8 approach.

Religious Fasting: Practices such as Ramadan urge fasting from sunrise until dusk.

Seasonal Eating

Many ancient tribes practiced seasonal eating, which involved ingesting foods that were only available at certain times of year. This approach valued the local ecosystem while also aligning dietary patterns with the earth's natural rhythms.

Health Benefits:

Nutrient-Rich Foods: Eating fruits and vegetables in season ensures that they are at their nutritious peak.

Diverse Diet: Seasonal eating promotes a diversified diet that contains a wide range of nutrients.

Sustainability: It encourages local agriculture while lowering the carbon impact associated with food transportation.

Examples:

Spring greens include dandelions, asparagus, and peas as they emerge in the spring.

Winter root vegetables include carrots, beets, and turnips, which store well during the colder months.

Whole foods

Ancient eating patterns frequently revolved around whole, unprocessed foods. Grains, fruits, vegetables, nuts, and seeds were the foundation of many cultures' meals, supplying critical nutrients without additions or preservatives.

Health Benefits:

Balanced Nutrition: Whole foods contain various vitamins, minerals, and antioxidants.

Weight Management: Foods in their original state are more satiating, which helps to regulate appetite.

Reduced Disease Risk: Whole-food diets have been linked to lower rates of chronic diseases such as heart disease and diabetes.

Examples:

Ancient Grains: Whole grains such as quinoa, farro, and spelt have been ingested for thousands of years.

Local veggies: Seasonal veggies and fruits high in fiber and antioxidants.

Recipes Inspired by Ancient Traditions.

Fermented cabbage salad (Sauerkraut)

Ingredients:

1 medium green cabbage.

One spoonful of sea salt

1 teaspoon of caraway seeds (optional)

Instructions:

Shred the cabbage finely and place it in a big bowl.

Sprinkle salt on the cabbage and knead it with your hands until it begins to exude juices.

If using caraway seeds, add them and pack the mixture tightly into a clean jar, making sure the liquid covers the cabbage.

Seal the jar and leave it ferment at room temperature for 1-4 weeks. Check the taste, and when it's sour enough, put it in the refrigerator.

Ginger Tea

Ingredients:

2 glasses of water.

1 tablespoon of fresh ginger, sliced

One teaspoon honey (optional)

Instructions:

Bring water to a boil in a saucepan.

Add the sliced ginger and boil for 10-15 minutes.

Strain into a cup and add honey if desired. Enjoy while still warm.

Mediterranean Grain Bowl

Ingredients:

One cup cooked farro or quinoa.

1 cup assorted seasonal veggies, such as bell peppers, zucchini, and tomatoes.

1/4 cup pitted and sliced olives.

1 tablespoon of olive oil.

1 tablespoon of lemon juice.

Add salt and pepper to taste.

Instructions:

In a mixing bowl, add the cooked farro or quinoa, mixed veggies, and olives.

Drizzle with olive oil and lemon juice, then season with salt and pepper.

Toss thoroughly and serve at room temperature.

Herbal Detox Soup

Ingredients:

4 cups veggie broth.

1 cup chopped kale.

1 cup chopped carrots.

1 cup of diced sweet potatoes.

1 teaspoon of turmeric powder.

1 teaspoon grated ginger.

Add salt and pepper to taste.

Instructions:

Heat the veggie broth in a big pot until it boils.

Add the carrots and sweet potatoes, and simmer until soft.

Stir in the kale, turmeric, ginger, salt, and pepper.

Simmer for 10 minutes and then serve warm.

Spiced Lentils Stew

Ingredients:

1 cup lentils, red or green

1 onion, chopped

2 garlic cloves, minced

1 teaspoon cumin.

1 teaspoon of coriander.

1 teaspoon of chili powder.

4 cups veggie broth.

Add salt and pepper to taste.

Instructions:

In a pot, cook the onion and garlic until tender.

Add the spices and simmer for another minute before adding the lentils and liquid.

Simmer for approximately 20-25 minutes, or until the lentils are soft. Season to taste, then serve.

Ancient dietary habits provide a wealth of wisdom, reminding us that the food we eat is inextricably linked to our health and well-being. Exploring these age-old customs can provide useful nutritional lessons that are relevant to our modern lifestyles.

Incorporating fermented foods, fasting, seasonal eating, and a focus on whole foods not only enriches our diets but also reconnects us with our ancestral roots. We may begin to alter our health one meal at a time by creating tasty meals based on these traditions. Embracing the past can lead to a healthier, more vibrant future by allowing us to respect the wisdom of those who came before us while also nurturing our bodies in the present.

Chapter 6: Mind-Body Connection.

Understanding the Importance of Mental Health in Ancient Healing

The old saying "mind over matter" resonates well in the context of holistic medicine. Ancient civilizations realized that the mind and body are interrelated systems that impact one another. This idea is more than just philosophical; it serves as the cornerstone for many traditional healing treatments throughout cultures.

In Traditional Chinese Medicine (TCM), Qi (or Chi) refers to the vital force that flows throughout the body. Blockages or imbalances in this energy can cause physical and emotional issues. Similarly, Ayurveda emphasizes the significance of mental clarity and emotional balance, claiming that mental well-being is critical to physical health. The ancient

Greeks, through Hippocrates' teachings, emphasised the impact of emotional moods on physical health, coining the term "psychosomatic" to characterize the mind's power over the body.

Contemporary medical research supports these ancient ideas. According to studies, stress and anxiety can emerge physiologically, resulting in heart disease, digestive issues, and chronic pain. In contrast, promoting mental health can improve immune function, reduce inflammation, and promote general well-being. The ancient practices we will look at in this chapter not only give useful approaches for improving mental health, but they also serve as reminders of the eternal wisdom that has led humanity for millenniums.

Ancient Cultures' Mindfulness and Meditation Practices

Meditation

Meditation is an ancient spiritual practice that originated in Buddhism and Hinduism. Meditation is really about developing awareness and inner calm. Ancient literature such as the Vedas and Buddhist sutras emphasize meditation's transformational power in obtaining inner peace and spiritual enlightenment.

Benefits:

Reduces stress and anxiety, resulting in better mental health.

Improves focus and concentration, hence promoting cognitive function.

Encourages emotional regulation, which helps people manage their reactions to difficulties.

Practical Exercise:

Basic Mindfulness Meditation:

Find a quiet place to sit comfortably.

Close your eyes and take some deep breaths.

Concentrate on your breath, noting each inhale and exhale.

When thoughts occur, gently recognize them and shift your focus back to your breath.

Practice for 5-10 minutes per day, gradually increasing the time as you get more comfortable.

Yoga

Yoga, which originated in ancient India, is more than simply physical postures; it is a whole discipline that combines the mind, body, and spirit. Ancient yogic works, such as Patanjali's Yoga Sutras, lay out the intellectual basis of yoga and its goal of leading a balanced, harmonious existence.

Benefits:

Improves physical flexibility and strength, which promotes overall fitness.

Mindfulness activities promote mental clarity and emotional stability.

Encourages a greater connection between the body and mind, which promotes self-awareness.

Practical Exercise:

Simple yoga sequence:

Mountain Pose (Tadasana): Stand tall with your feet together to ground yourself.

Downward Dog (Adho Mukha Svanasana): Bend forward with your hands on the ground and elevate your hips.

Warrior I (Virabhadrasana I): Step one foot back, bend the front knee, and raise the arms overhead.

Child's Pose (Balasana): Kneel and sit back on your heels, extending your arms forward and resting your forehead on the mat.

Hold each stance for 5-10 breaths while progressing through the pattern.

Breathwork

Ancient rituals from numerous cultures acknowledged the role of breath in healing. Pranayama (yogic breathing), for example, teaches practitioners to control their breath in order to regulate energy flow throughout the body. Similarly, Native American rituals frequently include breath as a technique of grounding and connecting with spirit.

Benefits:

It relieves stress by activating the parasympathetic nervous system.

Improves lung capacity and oxygenation, which benefits general health.

Encourages relaxation and emotional equilibrium.

Practical Exercise:

Breathing Technique: 4-7-8

Sit comfortably and close your eyes.

Inhale through your nose for a count of four.

Hold your breath for the count of seven.

Exhale slowly through your mouth for a count of eight.

Repeat 4-5 times, focusing on the rhythm of your breath.

Visualization

Visualization is an effective practice used in traditional therapeutic systems to realize intentions and increase mental clarity. This method entails envisioning a calm scenario or desired outcome, so using the mind's capacity to change reality.

Benefits:

Improves creativity and problem-solving skills.

Reduces anxiety by establishing a mental haven.

Facilitates goal achievement by instilling positive ideas.

Practical Exercise:

Guided Visualizations:

Find a peaceful area and close your eyes.

Take a few deep breaths and allow your body to relax.

Imagine a peaceful area, such as a beach, forest, or mountain.

Engage all of your senses: see colors, hear sounds, and touch textures.

Spend 5-10 minutes in this serene condition, letting your troubles go.

Practical Exercises to Improve Mental Health

Gratitude Journaling

Many ancient societies, including Native Americans and Buddhists, practiced thankfulness as a way to cultivate a healthy outlook. We can improve our general well-being by recognizing the positive aspects of our existence.

Exercise:

Set out a few minutes each day to jot down three things you are grateful for. Consider why these items are meaningful to you.

Nature Walks

Ancient methods frequently stressed the role of nature in healing. Connecting with the natural environment can relieve stress and increase mental clarity.

Exercise:

Spend time outside strolling in a natural atmosphere. Pay attention to the sights, sounds, and fragrances that around you. Allow yourself to be fully present, free of distractions.

Creative Expression

Artistic expression has traditionally been seen as a therapeutic technique. Ancient civilizations, like the Greeks and Indigenous tribes, recognized the healing value of creativity.

Exercise:

Participate in a creative endeavor like painting, drawing, or writing. Allow yourself to express your emotions and thoughts openly and without judgment.

Community Connection

Ancient societies put a high value on community and social relationships. Engaging with others promotes a sense of belonging and support, which is essential for mental health.

Exercise:

Participate in community events or join groups with similar interests. Develop relationships that promote your emotional well-being.

Digital Detox

The old idea of detaching from distractions is more applicable than ever in today's technology-driven environment. Taking a break from screens might improve brain clarity and reduce stress.

Exercise:

Set aside specified hours in the day to disconnect from digital devices. Use this time to meditate, read, or interact with loved ones.

The mind-body link is a powerful feature of ancient healing traditions that is still relevant in modern health approaches. Understanding the importance of mental well-being allows us to incorporate traditional cultural traditions into our daily lives, improving our total health.

Meditation, yoga, breathwork, and visualization are all disciplines that can help you create mindfulness and emotional balance. Furthermore, the practical exercises presented enable individuals to care for their mental health, developing a stronger connection to themselves and the world around them.

As we explore deeper into the ancient cures that might improve our health, let us embrace the timeless wisdom that leads us to holistic well-being, acknowledging that a healthy mind and body are inexorably intertwined. These activities enable us to handle the challenges of modern life with grace, resilience, and a stronger sense of purpose.

Chapter 7: Rituals and Remedies for Common Ails.

In today's fast-paced world, it is all too easy to ignore our bodies' soft whispers, particularly when it comes to common maladies such as headaches, stress, and stomach problems. However, ancient healing traditions provide a multitude of cures and rituals that not only address these common issues, but also restore balance and promote overall well-being. This chapter will look at numerous time-honored cures, including step-by-step instructions for preparation and use, as well as anecdotal success stories from people who have seen the significant advantages of these practices.

Solutions for Common Issues

1. Headaches

Headaches are a common ailment caused by a variety of circumstances, including stress, dehydration, and tension. Ancient traditions acknowledged the need of treating the underlying causes as well as the symptoms. Here are a few helpful remedies:

a. Peppermint Tea with Essential Oil

Peppermint has been utilized for ages due to its relaxing effects. The menthol in peppermint relaxes muscles and relieves headache discomfort.

Preparation:

Peppermint Tea:

Boil water, then pour it over a teaspoon of dried peppermint leaves.

Steep for 10 minutes, strain, and enjoy.

Peppermint Essential Oil:

Dilute a few drops of peppermint essential oil with a carrier oil (such as coconut or jojoba).

Gently massage the mixture into your temples and the back of your neck.

Anecdote:

Jessica, a graphic designer, frequently experienced stress headaches as a result of her long hours at the computer. She felt a lot better after she started drinking peppermint tea every day. "It became my go-to remedy," she explains. "The cool sensation on my temples was instantly soothing, and I felt more focused afterward."

b. Lavender inhalation

Lavender is well-known for its relaxing characteristics, making it an ideal choice for headache treatment.

Preparation:

Apply a few drops of lavender essential oil to a cotton ball.

Inhale deeply for several minutes, allowing the soothing aroma to fill your senses.

Anecdote:

David, a college student, learned about lavender inhalation during finals week. "I was stressed and had a pounding headache," he explains. "After inhaling lavender, I felt a wave of calm wash over me. It not only eased my headache but also helped me focus on my studies."

2. Stress

In today's environment, stress is a widespread problem that can harm both mental and physical health. Ancient healing techniques emphasize relaxation and awareness as effective stress relievers.

a. Ashwagandha Tea

Ashwagandha, an adaptogenic plant used in Ayurvedic medicine, is well-known for its stress-reducing qualities.

Preparation:

Bring water to a boil, then add one teaspoon of ashwagandha powder.

Simmer for 10 minutes, then drain and sweeten with honey as needed.

Anecdote:

Maria, a busy mother of three, turned to ashwagandha tea when she felt overwhelmed. "Within a few days of drinking it, I noticed a significant change in my mood. I felt more grounded and less anxious."

b. Mindful Breathing Ritual.

Mindful breathing is a simple yet effective technique that can be practiced anywhere. It soothes the mind and centers the spirit.

Preparation:

Find a quiet place to sit comfortably.

Inhale deeply through your nose for a count of four.

Hold your breath for a count of four.

Exhale slowly through your mouth for a count of six.

Repeat for a few minutes, focusing on your breathing.

Anecdote:

Eric, an entrepreneur, has included mindful breathing into his daily routine during high-pressure situations. "It's like a reset button for my mind," he says. "Whenever I feel overwhelmed, I take a moment to breathe deeply, and I emerge with clarity and calm."

3. Digestive Problems

Bloating and indigestion are two examples of digestive difficulties that can be exacerbated by stress and poor eating habits. Ancient traditions frequently make use of herbs and activities that promote healthy digestion.

a. Ginger Tea

Ginger is well-known for its digestive properties and has been utilized in many cultures for ages.

Preparation:

Slice fresh ginger root and boil in water for 10 minutes.

Strain and add lemon or honey to taste.

Anecdote:

Laura, who experienced periodic intestinal distress, received relief with ginger tea. "I used to rely on over-the-counter medications," she says with pride. "Now, a warm cup of ginger tea does wonders. It's comforting and effective."

b. Fermented foods

Including fermented foods in your diet can greatly enhance intestinal health. Kimchi, sauerkraut, and yogurt contain probiotics, which assist digestion.

Preparation:

Homemade sauerkraut:

Place a finely sliced head of cabbage in a big basin.

Sprinkle with salt and massage the cabbage to release its juices.

Pack the cabbage snugly into a jar, making sure it is submerged in the brine.

Seal the jar and leave it ferment at room temperature for 1-2 weeks.

Anecdote:

Tom, a health enthusiast, began making his own sauerkraut after learning about its health benefits. "I never realized how much my digestion would improve! It's become a staple in my diet," he jokes.

Step-by-Step Guides for Preparing and Using Remedies

Creating a herbal infusion:

Choose a herb (such as peppermint, ginger, or lavender).

Use either dried herbs or fresh leaves.

Boil the water and pour it over the herbs in a teapot or cup.

Steep for 5-15 minutes, depending on the herb and your desired strength.

Strain and serve warm or chilled.

Essential oil blends:

Choose your essential oils based on the intended effects (for example, lavender for relaxation and peppermint for headaches).

Add 3-5 drops of essential oil to a carrier oil.

Massage onto the troubled regions or disperse throughout your home to create a peaceful ambiance.

Homemade herbal capsules:

Collect your chosen plants in dry form.

Use empty capsules from health food stores.

Fill capsules with powdered herbs either by hand or with a capsule-filling machine.

Store in a cold, dark area and use as needed.

Creating A Relaxation Ritual:

Choose a peaceful area and assemble your ritual supplies (candles, incense, or relaxing music).

Set a timer for 10 to 20 minutes.

Light candles or incense and choose a comfortable seat.

Focus on your breath or use visualization techniques.

Anecdotal Success Stories from People Who Have Benefited

Emily's Transformation with Herbal Remedies:

After years of using prescription pain killers to treat her frequent headaches, Emily discovered the potential of herbal medicines. "I was skeptical at first," she tells me, "but after just a week of trying peppermint tea and lavender inhalation, I noticed a dramatic decrease in both the frequency and intensity of my headaches."

Jacob's Stress Relief Journey:

Jacob, a young professional, suffered from work-related stress, which led to insomnia. "I stumbled upon a mindfulness breathing exercise online and decided to give it a shot. It's incredible how just a few minutes of focused breathing can turn my day around. I feel more centered and can sleep better at night."

Nina's Gut Health Revival:

Nina had long struggled with digestive disorders, feeling bloated and uncomfortable after meals. She saw a considerable improvement after starting to drink ginger tea and eat fermented foods. "I never realized how much my digestion could change just by being more mindful of what I eat. It's empowering!"

The rituals and cures described in this chapter demonstrate the efficacy of ancient healing techniques in treating common diseases. By incorporating these time-honored cures into our daily lives, we can gain a better understanding of our bodies and improve our general health. The success stories of those who have adopted these techniques serve as a reminder that ancient wisdom still has transformative power in current times. As we traverse the complexity of health and wellness, let us rely on time-honored traditions that have nurtured mankind for generations, paving the way for holistic healing and vibrant health.

Chapter 8: The role of spirituality in healing

In ancient cultures, the delicate fabric of spirituality and health was woven together by threads of belief, ritual, and community. Spirituality has long been recognized as an essential component of holistic healing approaches, influencing not just physical health but also emotional and mental well-being. This chapter will look at how spirituality influences health in diverse ancient traditions, including practices such as prayer, rituals, and communal healing, as well as the critical importance of setting health intentions.

The Connection Between Spirituality and Health

Throughout history, many cultures have seen health as an integrated phenomena in which the physical body, mind, and spirit function in tandem. This comprehensive approach is critical for understanding how spirituality plays an important part in healing.

The ancient Greek idea of hygeia, named after the goddess of health, emphasized the necessity of balance and harmony in all aspects of life. Health was more than just the absence of disease; it was a condition of well-being that included bodily vigor, emotional stability, and spiritual congruence. Greek physicians, such as Hippocrates, emphasized the importance of a patient's mental and spiritual health, implying that emotional discomfort could lead to physical illness.

Similarly, traditional Chinese medicine (TCM) holds that health results from a balance of Qi (life force), yin and yang, and the interdependence of the body, mind, and spirit. TCM practitioners frequently combine meditation and mindfulness practices with acupuncture and herbal medicines, acknowledging the importance of spiritual well-being in obtaining overall health.

Spiritual Practices of Ancient Healing Traditions

1. Prayer

Prayer is one of the oldest kinds of spiritual practice, used across cultures to seek direction, comfort, and healing. In many indigenous cultures, prayer is more than just a call for divine intervention; it is also a means of connecting with nature and the universe.

Native American practices:

Prayer is typically an important part of Native American healing rituals. The medicine wheel, a symbol of healing and balance, integrates prayer as a means of connecting with the spiritual realm and seeking harmony with oneself and the natural world. Ceremonial prayers are said during healing ceremonies to invoke the spirits' guidance and support.

Christian Healing Traditions:

In Christianity, prayer is viewed as a direct method of communication with God. The New Testament is full with stories of Jesus curing people via prayer and faith. The sacrament of anointing the sick stresses the spiritual aspect of healing, as prayer is thought to elicit heavenly grace and aid in recovery.

2. Rituals

Rituals are powerful means of spiritual expression, frequently expressing a community's beliefs and ideals. These practices can foster a sense of belonging and connection with both the divine and other people.

Ancient Egyptian rituals:

In ancient Egypt, rituals were fundamental to the healing process. Priests, known as swnw, performed elaborate ceremonies involving chants, gifts, and the usage of holy symbols to elicit the gods' blessings on health. The rite of Opening the Mouth was done on mummies to ensure that the departed may enter the afterlife, emphasizing the need of spiritual health for both the living and the dead.

Hindu healing rituals:

Puja (worship) and yajna (fire offerings) are practices in Hinduism that evoke heavenly energy for healing. These rituals frequently involve the reading of sacred texts and mantras, which are said to channel spiritual energy and facilitate physical and mental healing. The ceremonial use of prasad, or blessed food, represents the interweaving of the spiritual and physical worlds.

3. Community Healing

The community aspect of spirituality in therapeutic activities creates a sense of belonging and support. Ancient cultures recognized the value of social relationships in maintaining health and frequently incorporated communal rituals into their healing procedures.

African Healing Traditions:

Many African cultures value community involvement in the healing process. Traditional healers, who are frequently regarded as spiritual leaders, lead the community in rituals that seek the ancestors' advice and help. This collaborative method not only treats the physical condition, but it also strengthens social relationships and promotes overall well-being.

Indigenous Australian healing circles:

Indigenous Australians participate in healing circles that emphasize community and storytelling. These circles provide an opportunity for people to share their struggles and receive support from others. Spirituality is integrated into these meetings through music, dancing, and the sharing of ancient wisdom, resulting in a powerful healing environment.

The Importance of Setting Health Goals

Setting intentions is a process that goes beyond old traditions and connects with modern wellness beliefs. Intentions serve as a guiding light, directing individuals' energy and efforts toward certain health outcomes. In ancient healing methods, setting intentions was frequently ritualized, emphasizing the importance of clarity and purpose in the healing process.

Power of Intention in Ayurveda:

In Ayurveda, intention is inextricably linked with the healing process. Ayurvedic practitioners frequently advise patients to set goals during treatments, whether they are for bodily healing, emotional balance, or spiritual growth. Sankalpa, or setting a resolution, is a typical process in which people express their intentions and connect their activities with the anticipated consequences.

Mindfulness and intention:

Modern mindfulness practices reflect the classical emphasis on intention setting. Mindfulness meditation allows people to set clear intentions for their practice, which promotes self-awareness and clarity. This intentionality can result in profound health changes as people become more aware of their bodies and emotions.

Practical Steps to Setting Intentions:

Clarity: Start by selecting particular health goals, such as physical health, emotional well-being, or spiritual development. To make these intentions more concrete, write them down.

Visualization: Take a moment to envision the desired result. Consider how fulfilling this intention would feel and what effect it would have on your life.

Create positive affirmations that reflect your aspirations. Repeat these affirmations every day to strengthen your dedication to your health goals.

Ritualization entails incorporating your aspirations into daily rituals, such as lighting a candle during meditation or constructing a vision board. These routines operate as concrete reminders of your aspirations.

Share your intentions with trusted friends and family members who can offer encouragement and support while you recuperate.

Spirituality plays a fundamental and diverse role in healing, including prayer, rituals, community healing, and intention-setting. Ancient traditions acknowledged the interdependence of the body, mind, and spirit, emphasizing that true healing requires addressing all components of oneself. As we delve into the wisdom of these traditions, we are reminded that spirituality provides not just a road to physical health, but also a greater knowledge of our place in the cosmos and our connections to others.

Incorporating spiritual traditions into our modern lives can enhance our recovery journeys by providing comfort, support, and a sense of purpose. Whether via prayer, social rituals, or the intentionality of our daily acts, we can use spirituality to build a holistic approach to health that values both our individual experiences and our shared humanity.

Chapter 9: Modern Application of Ancient Wisdom

In an age when the convergence of ancient wisdom and modern science opens up previously unheard-of healing possibilities, the revival of ancient remedies is no longer confined to the fringes of alternative medicine. This chapter delves into the use of ancient practices in modern healthcare through compelling case studies, the integration of traditional methods with conventional medicine, and the ethical issues surrounding the sourcing of natural remedies.

Ethical Concerns and Sustainability in Sourcing Natural Remedies

As interest in ancient treatments grows, ethical concerns about the procurement of natural cures have surfaced. If herbal goods and traditional medicine demand is not managed responsibly, it can strain local ecosystems and indigenous practices.

1. Ethical Sourcing Practices

Many practitioners are now highlighting the significance of procuring herbs and medicines responsibly. This involves assisting local farmers in cultivating herbs responsibly and campaigning for fair trade procedures that ensure local communities benefit from the commercialization of their traditional knowledge.

For example, the United Plant Savers promotes sustainable wildcrafting practices to safeguard native medicinal plants in North America. They hope to protect these plants for future generations by teaching consumers and practitioners about the environmental impact of herb harvesting.

2. Cultural sensitivity and respect for Indigenous knowledge.

Furthermore, integrating historical rituals requires cultural awareness and respect. For millennia, many indigenous tribes have preserved their knowledge of medicinal plants, and it is critical to recognize and compensate them for their contributions.

The World Health Organization (WHO) has underlined the significance of safeguarding traditional knowledge and involving indigenous groups in decision-making processes about their cultural traditions. This collaborative approach promotes a better awareness of the importance of ancient wisdom in modern healthcare while also protecting the rights of individuals who have maintained this information.

The modern uses of ancient knowledge demonstrate the enormous potential for incorporating old approaches into modern treatment. Case studies of practitioners such as Dr. Maoshing Ni and Dr. Deepak Chopra demonstrate how ancient treatments can complement contemporary medicine and provide comprehensive solutions to health problems.

As we traverse the complexity of healthcare in the twenty-first century, it is critical to maintain ethical standards when sourcing natural treatments and to honor the cultural heritage of historic healing traditions. By honoring the past and inventing for the future, we can create a healthcare paradigm that is truly integrative, sustainable, and representative of our common humanity.

The journey toward rejuvenating traditional remedies is about more than just recovery or therapy; it is about adopting a holistic approach to health that reflects the essence of who we are as individuals and as a society. This exploration will allow us to rediscover the transformative power of ancient wisdom, which will guide us to a happier, more balanced life.

Chapter 10: A Practical Guide to Beginning Your Healing Journey.

In today's fast-paced world, the pursuit of health and well-being can feel daunting. However, the ancient expertise of herbal treatments and holistic practices offers a diverse set of instruments for personal recovery. This chapter offers a practical guide to helping you start your healing journey, outlining how to establish a personal treatment plan, recommendations for sustainably procuring herbs and traditional items, and the value of keeping a notebook to track your progress and experiences.

Creating Your Personal Healing Plan

1. Assess your current health needs.

The first step in developing a personalized rehabilitation plan is to undertake a complete evaluation of your present health. This includes not only recognizing physical illnesses, but also taking into account your emotional and mental well-being.

Questions to consider:

What specific health difficulties do I currently have?

How do these concerns impact my daily life?

Do I have stress, worry, or other emotional difficulties?

What aspects of my health would I like to improve?

To learn more about your overall health, you could fill out a health assessment questionnaire or consult with a healthcare provider. This technique will assist you in determining your individual needs and setting attainable goals for your rehabilitation journey.

2. Identify Relevant Ancient Remedies.

Once you've examined your health needs, the following step is to look for traditional cures that can help with those specific issues. This could involve dietary changes, herbal medicines, meditation techniques, or other holistic approaches.

For example, if you have stomach troubles, you could check into:

Ginger is known for its digestive assist characteristics and ability to alleviate nausea.

Peppermint is commonly used to ease upset stomachs and enhance digestion.

If stress reduction is a priority, consider the following practices:

Mindfulness Meditation: Drawing on ancient Buddhist traditions, this practice can help you ground yourself and reduce worry.

Yoga is an ancient discipline that blends physical exercise, breath control, and meditation to promote total wellness.

Crafting Your Plan

When creating your healing plan, consider the following components:

Daily Rituals: Incorporate simple practices into your daily routine, such as morning herbal teas, evening meditation sessions, or conscious breathing exercises.

Nutrition: Create a diet plan that includes foods and herbs that support your recovery goals.

Physical Activity: To improve physical health and mental clarity, engage in frequent movement routines such as yoga, walking, or tai chi.

3. Set realistic goals and milestones.

When developing your healing plan, it is critical to identify realistic goals and milestones. Remember that mending is typically a gradual process that demands patience and perseverance.

Considerations for goal setting:

Define your short- and long-term goals. Short-term goals could include drinking herbal tea three times per week, and long-term goals could entail considerable lifestyle changes.

Monitor your development on a regular basis and celebrate little triumphs. Each step forward represents a victory!

4. Seek guidance from practitioners.

Consider speaking with practitioners who specialize in the ancient healing systems you want to investigate. This could include herbalists, acupuncturists, and Ayurvedic practitioners. They can offer personalized counsel and support as you embark on your healing journey.

Tips for Purchasing Herbs and Traditional Products Responsibly

As you add ancient medicines into your healing regimen, it's critical to obtain your herbs and goods properly. Here are some tips to help you:

1. Choose Quality Over Quantity.

When purchasing herbs and traditional items, emphasis quality. Look for trusted suppliers who follow sustainable harvesting procedures and offer organic, non-GMO products. Quality herbs are more effective and good to your health.

2. Support Local and Sustainable Sources.

Whenever possible, look for local herbalists, farmers' markets, or community-supported agriculture (CSA) programs. This not only benefits local economies, but it also assures that the herbs you use are fresh and ethically sourced.

3. Educate yourself on sourcing practices.

Be aware of the source processes of the herbs you wish to utilize. Investigate whether the plants are harvested sustainably and if the company promotes fair trade practices. Organizations such as United Plant Savers and the American Herbalists Guild provide tools to assist people make informed decisions.

4. Understand Indigenous knowledge.

When sourcing traditional remedies, remember to respect indigenous cultures' cultural heritage and knowledge. Seek to grasp the context and significance of the plants you're employing, and avoid appropriating their traditions without proper acknowledgment and respect.

Keeping a journal to document progress and experiences

Keeping a journal during your healing process is an effective tool for self-reflection and progress tracking. Here's how to efficiently keep a journal:

1. Document your experiences.

Keep a regular record of your experiences with the remedies you're utilizing, including any changes in your physical, emotional, or mental health. This can help you figure out what works best for you and change your strategy accordingly.

Suggested journal prompts:

What cures did I try today, and how did I feel afterwards?

What challenges did I face, and how did I overcome them?

What fresh insights have I gotten into my health?

2. Reflect on your goals.

Review your goals on a regular basis and track your progress. Reflecting on your path can bring significant insights and strengthen your dedication to your treatment plan.

3. Celebrate Milestones.

Don't forget to celebrate your achievements! Recognizing your accomplishments, no matter how modest, can improve motivation and remind you of the beneficial changes you are implementing.

4. Seek support from others.

Consider sharing your journal with a trusted friend or healthcare provider who understands your path. They can offer encouragement and comments, making the process more rewarding.

Beginning your healing journey with ancient medicines is an empowering experience that allows you to reconnect with your body, mind, and soul. You can create a holistic approach to health and well-being by developing a personal healing plan tailored to your specific needs, obtaining herbs responsibly, and keeping a journal to document your progress.

As you embrace the knowledge of ancient traditions, keep in mind that healing is an individual path. It necessitates patience, self-compassion, and an eagerness to learn and adapt. Allow this chapter to guide you as you begin your journey toward a better, more vibrant existence.

On this trip, you will discover not only physical healing, but also a deep connection to ancient practices that have stood the test of time. As you combine traditional traditions with current awareness, you may gain a better understanding of yourself and the world around you, paving the way for holistic well-being that benefits all aspects of your life.

Conclusion: Revitalizing Ancient Wisdom for Modern Wellness.

As we stand at the confluence of traditional wisdom and modern science, it becomes evident that our ancestors' practices and medicines have enormous promise for improving our health. The renewed interest in traditional healing practices reflects a deeper human desire for connection, balance, and holistic health in a society that frequently feels fragmented and chaotic. This conclusion highlights the necessity of conserving and appreciating these historic practices, encourages readers to embrace their particular health journeys, and advocates for active participation in the continuous exploration and exchange of information.

Preserving and Honouring Ancient Healing Traditions

Ancient healing traditions contain insight that demonstrates humanity's endurance and adaptation throughout history. Cultures all throughout the world have created complicated knowledge systems based on observation, experience, and a strong connection to nature. These traditions not only give cures for diseases, but they also provide light on the interdependence of body, mind, and spirit.

As we implement these practices into our life, we must remember the sources of this knowledge and the cultures from which it arose. Preservation efforts are critical to preserve the authenticity of these traditions. This involves:

Education and Awareness: Understanding the historical background and cultural relevance of ancient healing traditions allows us to better appreciate their contributions. Learning about the concepts that govern these traditions enables us to better respectfully incorporate them into our own lives.

Sustainable Practices: When seeking herbs and medicines, it is critical to do so in a manner that respects the environment and the communities that rely on these resources. Supporting sustainable harvesting practices helps to maintain biodiversity while also empowering indigenous populations.

Intercultural Respect: Engaging with historic healing practices needs respect for those who have passed down this knowledge through centuries. It is critical to avoid cultural appropriation by acknowledging and appreciating the contributions of all cultures.

By advocating the preservation of historic healing methods, we contribute to a larger conversation about health and wellness that spans time and place. By doing so, we build a stronger feeling of community, empathy, and interconnectedness.

Embracing Personal Health Journeys

Each person's health path is unique, influenced by their own experiences, beliefs, and circumstances. Ancient healing methods offer a broad toolkit that may be customized to address a variety of needs. Here are some methods to encourage readers to investigate and appreciate their personal health journeys:

Cultivating Curiosity: Approach health and wellbeing with an open mind and a sense of adventure. Explore the broad realm of ancient treatments, dietary regimens, and meditation techniques. Each step into this realm brings new perspectives and opportunity for personal development.

Empower yourself via knowledge: Learn about the healing powers of plants, nutritional options, and holistic practices. The more you understand, the more confident you will be in making informed health decisions.

Listen to your body's messages and responses. Integrating ancient techniques is more than just following a recipe; it is about listening to your own demands. To manage your recovery process, follow your body's cues.

Seeking Community: Surround yourself with people who share your interest in holistic health and ancient healing practices. Participating in a supportive community can offer motivation, inspiration, and a sense of belonging.

Being Open to Change: Recognize that healing is a dynamic process that may require trial and error. Be willing to change your approach as you learn what resonates with you.

Call to Action: Share your experiences and continue learning.

As you begin your healing path, know that you are not alone. Countless others are delving into ancient wisdom and discovering their own paths to wellbeing. Here is a call to action for readers to share their experiences and keep learning:

Document Your Journey: Keep track of your experiences with ancient cures, dietary changes, and holistic practices. Reflecting on your success not only increases self-awareness, but it also helps you understand what genuinely works for you.

Engage with friends, family, and social media communities to share your knowledge and experiences. Your experience may inspire others to follow their own paths to wellbeing, creating a ripple effect of healing and connection.

Participate in Workshops and Events: Look for local or online workshops focused on ancient healing traditions. Engaging with experts and practitioners can help you gain a better grasp of health issues and broaden your toolkit.

Continue Learning: Embrace lifelong learning by studying books, podcasts, and videos about ancient healing methods. Every new piece of information broadens your understanding and improves your capacity to navigate your health journey.

Advocate for Holistic Health: Become an advocate for incorporating ancient wisdom into modern wellness techniques. Support projects that promote holistic health, natural treatments sourced sustainably, and cultural heritage preservation with respect.

In a culture that frequently favors quick fixes and technical advances, resurrecting traditional knowledge for modern wellbeing provides a welcome alternative. Our forefathers' habits encourage us to slow down, reconnect with ourselves and environment, and adopt a holistic approach to health. By maintaining and honoring these traditions, we recognize the important insights they provide and pave the path for a healthier, more balanced tomorrow.

Remember that every stage of your healing path is significant. Your dedication to researching ancient medicines, appreciating their origins, and sharing your findings helps to weave a common tapestry of wellness that spans time and culture. Together, we can promote a better understanding of health, build resilience, and appreciate the diversity of life.

May your path be filled with discovery, empowerment, and connection as you embrace the ancient wisdom with the potential to transform modern wellness.

The end

www.ingramcontent.com/pod-product-compliance
Lightning Source LLC
Chambersburg PA
CBHW070146230526
45471CB00002B/543